50 THINGS TO KNOW ABOUT BECOMING A MEDICAL DOCTOR

Tong (Toni) Liu, MD

50 Things to Know About Becoming a Medical Doctor Copyright © 2019 by CZYK Publishing LLC. All Rights Reserved.

All rights reserved. No part of this book may be reproduced in any form or by any electronic or mechanical means including information storage and retrieval systems, without permission in writing from the author. The only exception is by a reviewer, who may quote short excerpts in a review.

The statements in this book are of the authors and may not be the views of CZYK Publishing or 50 Things to Know.

Cover designed by: Ivana Stamenkovic
Cover Image: https://pixabay.com/photos/stethoscope-Medical-health-doctor-2617701/

CZYK Publishing Since 2011.

50 Things to Know

Lock Haven, PA
All rights reserved.
ISBN: 9781673554861

50 THINGS TO KNOW ABOUT BECOMING A MEDICAL DOCTOR

BOOK DESCRIPTION

What is it like in Medical School? What should I expect from choosing Medicine as a career? How do I decide if it's right for me? If you answered yes to any of these questions then this book is for you...

"50 Things to Know About Becoming a Medical Doctor" by Dr. Toni Liu offers an approach to understanding the Medical training path. Most books on Medical School tell you how to study and prepare for tests and tasks. Although there's nothing wrong with that, they don't talk about how mentally difficult and rigorous Medical training will be, and how best to prepare yourself for the tough journey ahead.

In these pages you'll discover the truth about training to become a doctor. This book will help you prepare yourself if that's the path you choose.

By the time you finish this book, you will know all about the Medical training path, what to expect, and whether it's right for you. So grab YOUR copy today. You'll be glad you did.

TABLE OF CONTENTS

BOOK DESCRIPTION
TABLE OF CONTENTS
DEDICATION
ABOUT THE AUTHOR
INTRODUCTION
1. Learn The Logistics And Time-frame
2. Medical School Is Hands-On
3. You Can Customize Your Education
4. Know What Residency Is
5. Understand The Process of Applying
6. Understand "The Match"
7. Medical School Spots And Residency Spots Do Not Match Up
8. Because Residency Spots Are Limited, They Are Usually Short-Staffed
9. Consider Combined Programs
10. Understand The Financial Burden
11. Consider International Medical Schools
12. Start Exploring Early
13. Ask Doctors Tough Questions, Don't Be Shy
14. Speak To Many Different Types of Doctors
15. Even Ask Doctors Who Don't See Patients
16. Don't Forget About Non-Clinical Doctors

17. If You Like Research, Consider An MD-PhD Degree
18. You Can Take Time Off
19. Learn About The Worst So You Can Prepare
20. Ask About And Imagine The Best
21. Think About What Way of Helping Feels Most Gratifying To You
22. Try To Figure Out Why That Way Feels Gratifying
23. Think About Your Skills And Personality In Regards To This Field
24. But Keep An Open Mind
25. Don't Do It For The Money
26. Look At Other Healthcare Options
27. Think About How Much Autonomy You Want
28. Assess Your Test-Taking Skills
29. Ask Yourself Honestly, "Do I Enjoy Lifelong Learning?"
30. Ask Yourself, "Can I Handle Competition?"
31. Ask Yourself, "Do I Fit In With These People?"
32. Be Prepared To Work Very Long Hours
33. Assess Your Time-Management Skills
34. Be Prepared To Work Odd, Irregular Hours
35. Check How You Handle Sleep Deprivation
36. Be Aware Of High Malpractice Rates

37. You Will Likely Spend More Time With A Computer, Than With Patients
38. Medical Documentation Is Unnecessarily Complex
39. You Will Not Have As Much Autonomy As You Think
40. You Will Have More Control Over Your Schedule Once You Fully Complete The Path
41. You Can Work in Academic Or Private Practice
42. You Can Also Do A Fellowship For Even More Training
43. Mental Health Issues Affect At Least One-Third Of All Doctors
44. The System Is Slow to Change
45. Any Wavering Is Seen As Weakness
46. Asking For Help Is Extremely Difficult Due To Stigma
47. Going To One's Own Appointments Is Difficult
48. Medicine Is An Occupational Risk Factor For Suicide
49. You Don't Have to Suffer Silently
50. Check In With Yourself Often

Other Helpful Resources:

50 Things to Know

DEDICATION

To my family, friends, and all my brave colleagues who ever have, ever will, or ever thought about going through the tough journey of Medical training.

ABOUT THE AUTHOR

Tong (Toni) Liu is a Chinese-American, Board-Certified, licensed Family Medicine physician with a background in Obstetrics and Gynecology. Having experienced two Residencies, she can speak to the unique challenges of both primary care and surgical fields.

She ultimately decided to leave traditional Medicine behind and made a huge career shift into the more creative fields she had always yearned for (cartooning, writing, coaching, and teaching) while traveling the world. She does do a bit of Telemedicine and Locum Tenens work as a mental health and women's rights advocate.

You can find her at her blog https://LTnomad.com and on her Facebook page LTnomad.

INTRODUCTION

"In an endless sea of overindulgence, find time to indulge in something worthwhile and make an informed, educated decision for yourself. What matters to you in here, will matter to you out there."

— K.A. Linde

Many people dream of becoming doctors. Doctors are needed in this world; there is a shortage. They do important, rewarding work, and are highly respected. Medicine is almost a default profession that almost everyone considers at some point or another. But that doesn't mean it is right for everybody.

Many don't know much about the actualities of the process, the life they will have afterwards, or how to decide if it's the right path for them. Becoming a doctor is a long road, with many challenging twists and turns, and lots of jumping through hoops. What many do not know is, that it's a highly risky job, not just to the patients, but to the doctors themselves.

Growing up in an Asian family, in which both parents were doctors, I felt pressured to become a doctor even more intensely. My journey has been a long one, of getting lost and finding my true self again. Had I known what I now know about the Medical path, I don't think I would have chosen it.

I wrote this book hoping to give others as much information as possible so they can make the best decisions for themselves and each of their unique situations. I hope no one will ever again step into this field blindly, or wish they had more information earlier.

<u>Note:</u> This book is about the Medical training path in the United States; I do not have a good enough firsthand understanding of other countries' systems to speak about them. I did however do month-long shadowing rotations in China, Taiwan, and Japan, and can say cultures and practices vary widely between countries. For example, those countries usually saw more patients in a day than the U.S. (closer to 40 patients per day instead of 20).

1. LEARN THE LOGISTICS AND TIME-FRAME

There are some exceptions, but the usual path to becoming a doctor involves 4 years of undergraduate education at a College/University, 4 years of Medical School, then at least 3 years of training in a "Residency program." The Residency training depends on what type of doctor you become, or specialty you choose. For example, a Pediatrician's (children's doctor) training is 3 years, whereas a Neurosurgeon's training is 7 years long. Of note, podiatrists (foot doctors) and dentists have their own special schools and do not go through Medical School.

When you graduate Medical School, you will no longer be a "doctor-in-training" or "student doctor." You will have gotten your MD (Medical Doctor) or DO (Doctor of Osteopathic Medicine) degree and will be considered a full doctor, however you will not be able to see patients on your own until you have completed sufficient Residency training. During Residency, you are known as a "Resident doctor," and after you graduate Residency, you will be an

"Attending doctor," the most senior kind, and able to practice Medicine fully independently. If you choose to further specialize and gain more specialized skills, you may opt to do a "Fellowship" after Residency, which can last 1-3 years.

What many people do not know is that licensing and Board Certification are two different processes. A doctor can get a license to practice Medicine after only 1 or 2 years of Residency training, depending on the state. But to become Board-Certified, you need to fully finish and graduate from a Residency program, to become eligible to sit for the Board exams ("Board-Eligible"). There are some people who drop out of Residency to start practicing, for various reasons, or sometimes their Residency programs shut down or lose accreditation. Your job options are more limited if you are not Board-Certified, so most people try to finish Residency if possible.

50 Things to Know

Specialty	Median Compensation	Years of Residency Training
Neurosurgery	$548,186	6*
Orthopedic surgery	$476,083	5*
Radiology	$438,115	5
Radiation oncology	$413,518	5
Plastic Surgery	$388,929	6
Anesthesiology	$366,640	4
ENT	$365,171	5
Dermatology	$350,627	4
General Surgery	$340,000	5*
Ophthalmology	$325,384	4
Obstetrics and gynecology	$294,190	4
Pathology	$285,173	4
Emergency medicine	$267,293	3-4
Physical medicine & rehabilitation	$236,800	4
Neurology	$236,500	4
Psychiatry	$208,462	4
Internal medicine	$205,441	3
Pediatrics	$202,832	3
Family medicine	$197,655	3

*an additional 1-2 years of research may be required at some programs

Source: *The Ultimate Guide to Choosing a Medical Specialty*, 2013, Brian Freeman MD

2. MEDICAL SCHOOL IS HANDS-ON

The first year or two of Medical School is classroom-style, as you learn, study, and take exams. But a big part of being a doctor is learning clinical skills and gaining experience on the job. You will see mock patients and be observed on your skills of gathering information, building connections with, and examining patients. You will also help out teams of Resident and Attending doctors in hospitals ("Inpatient" settings because patients typically stay overnight), clinics ("Outpatient" settings), schools, and other settings. Be prepared for learning in many different forms. You will never see a patient fully alone – you will report to a Resident doctor, Attending doctor, or both.

You can really help other doctors out and contribute to the team since you will have more time than they do to spend with patients, since you will have fewer responsibilities and fewer patients assigned to you. (For example, in the hospital setting, of all the hospitalized patients the team cares for, the average Resident doctor takes care of 7-10 patients per day, but a Medical Student is typically assigned only 1-3 patients.)

3. YOU CAN CUSTOMIZE YOUR EDUCATION

As a Medical Student, you do rotations through hospitals, clinics, and other facilities, covering several Medical fields to help you decide which one to go into for yourself. There are mandatory ones that everyone rotates through, such as Surgery, Pediatrics, Internal Medicine, and Obstetrics & Gynecology. But you also have flexibility to choose other areas to explore, called "Electives," and some schools even offer international opportunities. Definitely speak with your advisors to learn about all your options. You can even propose a new kind of rotation if there is someone or some specific niche field you are really interested in. You may also be asked to do research, either during the year or the summers, and some students even take a full year to dedicate to research. Of note, every Medical School is different, but typically there is only one summer break of the entire curriculum, in between 1st and 2nd year.

4. KNOW WHAT RESIDENCY IS

At the end of Medical School, you receive your MD (Medical Doctor) or DO (Doctor of Osteopathic Medicine) degree. But the amount of clinical experience you had in Medical School isn't enough for you to start seeing patients by yourself. Thus you need to go through a Residency training program, where you work as a junior doctor, overseen by senior doctors. You get a fixed salary, ranging from $50,000-70,000, but this unfortunately translates to a meager hourly wage since you sometimes have to work 80 hours per week. The first year of any Residency is called "Intern Year," not to be confused with internships done before Medical School or in other job fields.

5. UNDERSTAND THE PROCESS OF APPLYING

For Medical School, you must take the MCAT test (a standardized test such as the SAT, but specifically for people going into Medicine) and apply and interview like most other school and job applications. You must also make sure that you completed the necessary "Pre-Requisite Classes" in College/University, such as Physics, Organic Chemistry, and Biology.

You can be accepted to multiple schools, and you can decide which one to go to. Since they are so competitive, it's advised to apply to many, at least 15, to make sure you have a good chance of getting a spot. Most recent data shows that over 50,000 people apply for Medical School, but only 500 (1%) or so are accepted. There is a shortage of Medical Schools all over the world, and an even bigger shortage of Residency training programs. Every year, there are more and more applicants as well, so it will only become even more competitive.

6. UNDERSTAND "THE MATCH"

For Residency programs, the application process is very different. You still apply to and interview at as many programs as you want, but you have to rank them in your order of preference and submit them to a computer system called "The Match." This system's algorithm then factors in your preferences and each program's preferences to create the final result. You get "Matched" to 1 and only 1 Residency program, and you only have 2 choices – to go or not to go. If you decide not to go, you will have to re-do the entire process again next year, and it may look bad on your record that you had a gap year.

7. MEDICAL SCHOOL SPOTS AND RESIDENCY SPOTS DO NOT MATCH UP

Unfortunately, the current system does not quite make sense - there are far more Medical School spots than there are Residency spots. As a result, some Medical Students do not "Match" because their top Residency programs preferred other candidates for their limited spots. On "Match Day," which is always a Friday in March of the 4th year of Medical School, you first find out if you "Matched" at all on that Monday. If you did not, you have the option to "Scramble," meaning to reach out to any programs that still have leftover openings. They may not even have been programs you interviewed at or considered before, but it is better to have any Residency program than to have none at all (the stigma of the "Un-Matched" status).

8. BECAUSE RESIDENCY SPOTS ARE LIMITED, THEY ARE USUALLY SHORT-STAFFED

For various reasons, including funding, work volume, and availability of certain training experiences, Residency spots are limited, and so they are almost always short-staffed. They can only accommodate a certain number of trainees since they want to make sure every person gets an adequate hands-on education. Surgical specialties are smaller for this reason, because each surgeon needs to do a certain number of surgical cases to be considered fully trained, and some procedures are quite rare (for example, an "open" surgery, where doctors make a large incision, since nowadays there are many less invasive ways to perform surgeries, using camera scopes and robots).

9. CONSIDER COMBINED PROGRAMS

There are some programs that combine undergraduate and Medical School educations. Some of these are as short as 6 years, if you are looking to save time. However, the downside of these programs is that you have to decide on Medicine as a career early on, in high school. Many people may not have had enough life experiences yet to make such a huge decision. Many do not yet have a solid understanding of who they truly are and what they truly want, their strengths and weaknesses, among many other factors.

10. UNDERSTAND THE FINANCIAL BURDEN

In the United States, 4 years of Medical School tuition costs around $250,000 (a quarter-million dollars)! Many people do not have this kind of money so they have to take out student loans, which is a very unforgiving system. The loans will increase by about 7% every year, and they will still be there even if you declare bankruptcy, unlike other debts. If you also have loans from College/University, your debt will be even higher. Many doctors are still paying back their debts in their 40s.

11. CONSIDER INTERNATIONAL MEDICAL SCHOOLS

Since U.S. Medical Schools are so costly, some people go to schools in other countries where the tuition is cheaper, such as the Caribbean. These schools may be less competitive and easier to get accepted into, as well. The downside, however is that they usually have a harder time getting into Residency programs because international Medical Schools are not as reputable as Medical Schools within the U.S. You can consider schools that have a partnership with certain Residency programs, however.

12. START EXPLORING EARLY

Start exploring what it means to be a doctor as early as you can – in high school, or middle school even. Volunteering at a hospital is not necessarily accurate since they may have you do unrelated tasks such as desk work, answering calls, or fetching water for patients. Try to ask to shadow the doctors themselves directly. Be aware and respectful that doctors will usually have Medical Students or

Residents with them already, and that it may be too overwhelming for the patients if you join the team in the room as well.

13. ASK DOCTORS TOUGH QUESTIONS, DON'T BE SHY

Ask the doctors you shadow specific questions, even if they are very direct or blunt. Ask them if they're happy. Ask them if they would have chosen this same path if they could do it all over again. Ask them about anything they wish they had known sooner or done differently.

14. SPEAK TO MANY DIFFERENT TYPES OF DOCTORS

There are so many specialties within Medicine, and so many directions you can go. The lives and realities of each field are very different. When you ask doctors questions, try to ask as many different types of doctors as possible. A Surgeon's life is very different from that of a General Practitioner/Primary Care Physician's. Some specialties work regular 9-5 office hours, but others are "on call" and have to work irregular shifts, or at times even 24-hour shifts. For example, an Obstetrician (doctor who delivers babies) has to come in to deliver babies at any time of day or night. Other doctors are on "home call," meaning they must be available to answer patients' telephone calls at any time of day or night, but they may not have to leave their homes. A doctor can be on "home call" for long stretches, such as a full week or two.

15. EVEN ASK DOCTORS WHO DON'T SEE PATIENTS

There are types of doctors who don't directly see or talk to patients. These fields, such as Radiology (doctors who read x-rays and other images) or Pathology (doctors who look at specimens from patients under microscopes), are still crucial to healthcare. If you are shy or introverted, don't forget to consider these options.

16. DON'T FORGET ABOUT NON-CLINICAL DOCTORS

Then there are jobs in which doctors don't take care of patients at all. These are called "non-clinical jobs." These doctors still use the information they learned in Medical School, but for more behind-the-scenes roles, such as a consultant who reviews malpractice cases, or a public health administrator. There are not as many non-clinical jobs as there are clinical jobs, however. If you know you want a non-clinical job, you sometimes may not need to finish a full Residency training program since those are geared for those who want to practice Medicine clinically.

17. IF YOU LIKE RESEARCH, CONSIDER AN MD-PHD DEGREE

There is a combined MD-PhD degree for those who enjoy research. It is usually 6 years long, instead of the typical 4 years of Medical School. You can also add on a Masters of Public Health (MPH) degree to an MD/DO degree as well.

18. YOU CAN TAKE TIME OFF

Don't forget that you can also take up to a few years off before or during Medical School if you want to gain some work experience, explore research, try an internship, study for a specific test, or just take a break. Some combined programs even allow this. For example, my program (The Warren Alpert Medical School of Brown University) allowed up to 2 years off between College/University and Medical School, though I did not take advantage of it.

It is generally frowned upon to take time off between Medical School and Residency. Usually this is not the student's choice, because they did not "Match" into a Residency program and have to wait a full year before they can re-apply. There is only one Match each year, in the spring (see #6).

It is most difficult to take a pause during Residency, since you are counted on for work in an already short-staffed system (see #8).

After Residency graduation, some people take time off as well, but any gaps longer than 6 months will

...cluded and explained in any future ... for Medical licenses.

In general, people take time off for different reasons, and they are all valid. Some companies and agencies may ask about the gaps in your resume though. Just be prepared to talk about them.

Take the time that you need so you can feel balanced and confident about your decisions.

19. LEARN ABOUT THE WORST SO YOU CAN PREPARE

Ask doctors what are the toughest parts of their jobs. What was their most difficult experience(s)? Now imagine yourself in their shoes, in that same situation, and see how you feel. Do you freeze up, or do you rise up to that immense responsibility? Imagining the worst, even as a mental exercise, counts as practice, and will make future similar situations easier to handle. However, if it is very traumatic or difficult for you, it is a sign of strength, rather than weakness, to know yourself well enough to pivot or change your trajectory.

20. ASK ABOUT AND IMAGINE THE BEST

Don't forget to ask doctors about the best parts of their jobs. What do they find most rewarding about their careers? What were their best days like? Imagine yourself in their shoes and notice the feelings that arise for you.

21. THINK ABOUT WHAT WAY OF HELPING FEELS MOST GRATIFYING TO YOU

Not everyone needs to know what type of doctor they want to become, but it's worth thinking about and imagining. Do you like to fix problems quickly? Do you like emergency situations where you literally save someone's life? Do you like to build long-term relationships with patients and see them over the course of their and your lives?

22. TRY TO FIGURE OUT WHY THAT WAY FEELS GRATIFYING

Is there a specific group of people you most feel for and want to help, such as children or the elderly? Is it because a loved one went through a similar problem? The more you know the "why" behind your interest in a particular field, the better you'll be able to keep pushing on when things get hard.

23. THINK ABOUT YOUR SKILLS AND PERSONALITY IN REGARDS TO THIS FIELD

You should look critically at yourself and assess whether you are a good fit for the field you have in mind. If you are squeamish about blood, then surgery probably isn't for you. If your mind goes blank in emergency situations, then working in an emergency department or a labor and delivery floor probably isn't for you.

24. BUT KEEP AN OPEN MIND

Even if you know exactly what type of doctor you want to become, your interests may change as you go through the process. That's okay. For some people (including me), they even realize they want to change halfway or towards the end of one Residency program; it's not too late to change even then! You can use The Match again, or use other special websites to facilitate this (you can find these in the Resources section at the end).

For me, I changed halfway through a 4-year Obstetrics & Gynecology program to Family Medicine. I did receive some credit for my previous 2 full years of training and was able to graduate my Family Medicine program in 2.25 years instead of 3 years. Each program is different, however. For example, another Family Medicine program I was considering only gave me 4 months of credit, instead of 9 months. Each specific situation will be different. I did not use The Match again; I directly emailed the Program Directors of the Residency programs after hearing they had openings.

This isn't talked about as much, but many people change Residencies, either within the same field, or into a different field. It is nothing to be ashamed of. Some people may not have gotten adequate exposure and information to a certain field from Medical School, and others change because of geographic, family, or even personal reasons such as wanting a better work-life balance. Most recent statistics show that only 70% of Residents graduate from the same/original Residency program they started in!

25. DON'T DO IT FOR THE MONEY

The crazy costs of Medical tuition pressure many people into choosing specialties with higher salaries. There is a huge range of salaries depending on the type of field. For example, the average Pediatrician (children's doctor) makes $200,000, whereas a Dermatologist (skin doctor) makes $350,000. As tempting as the money may be, don't let it drastically affect your decisions. At the end of the day, pick a specialty of Medicine that you enjoy for a reason other than the pay.

26. LOOK AT OTHER HEALTHCARE OPTIONS

If you enjoy science and want to help people as a healthcare worker, try to avoid having tunnel vision. Being a doctor isn't the only way to help patients. You can be a Physician's Assistant (PA), Nurse Practitioner (NP), Nurse Anesthetist (CRNA), Physical Therapist (DPT), Emergency Medical Technician (EMT), and much, much more. These training paths are shorter and less expensive, and can have the same satisfaction and even day-to-day life as a physician's, and make comparable salaries as well.

They may also have unique advantages. For example, a PA can change specialties at any time, including assisting with surgeries, if you are someone who gets bored easily and want to try out several different fields. Also, financially comparing the average debts of Mid-Level Providers vs. doctors and considering how quickly the debt grows (7% each year), one study found that doctors will only catch up to them in their 40s.

27. THINK ABOUT HOW MUCH AUTONOMY YOU WANT

Do you like being in charge? Many Mid-Level providers (PAs and NPs) practice Medicine independently. Even though they need to have a "Supervising" physician's name as a co-signer on their decisions, there are many places where they practice independently and only consult the Supervising physician over the phone if they have questions. For some people, they don't mind having someone to consult, or even find comfort in it. For others, they want and need to make all the decisions all by themselves, but there is also more responsibility involved.

28. ASSESS YOUR TEST-TAKING SKILLS

The Medical path is full of tests, and they will never stop. Even after finishing all your training, you will need to re-take your Board Certification exams every 10 years, until you retire. The Board exams are held only once or twice a year. If you are not a strong test-taker, be sure to practice extra to hone those skills. You will have some chances to re-take tests, but the failed tests will always show up on your record, which can bar you from certain opportunities. After the MCAT, every Medical trainee will need to take licensing exams, usually USMLE Step 1, Step 2, and Step 3. These standardized tests are quite long, usually 8 hours. Step 3 is a 2-day exam, but those days do not have to be back-to-back anymore.

There is also Step 2 Clinical Skills which is a recorded observational exam of you conducting interviews and examining mock patients. Of note, there are only 5 facilities in the entire country that offer Step 2 Clinical Skills, so Medical Students will have to schedule specific dates and travel to those cities (Atlanta, GA, Chicago, IL, Houston, TX, Los Angeles, CA, and Philadelphia, PA).

Board certifications vary by specialty. Some specialties only require sitting for a Written Board exam (all multiple-choice questions). Others, such as Emergency Medicine and Surgery, require passing an Oral Board exam (free responses), and again, this is only offered in certain facilities at certain times, usually only once a year.

29. ASK YOURSELF HONESTLY, "DO I ENJOY LIFELONG LEARNING?"

Medicine is constantly changing as we make new discoveries, and you need to stay up to date. You will always need to keep reading articles, books, and journals, and studying to keep your skills sharp. If you are someone who does not like learning, reading, or remaining flexible to new changes, this may not be the right path for you.

30. ASK YOURSELF, "CAN I HANDLE COMPETITION?"

They say doctors make up the top 1% of the population. Medical School is one of the most competitive schools out there, not just to get into, but also to get out of. This road will be intense and your grades may be affected by how well others perform (this is called a "curved" scoring method). You may also have colleagues who are very competitive and try to outshine you by racing to answer a question, for example. Some Medical Schools and Residency programs are more competitive than others, but the overall culture of the Medical training path leans more towards competition rather than collaboration, since there are just so few available spots.

31. ASK YOURSELF, "DO I FIT IN WITH THESE PEOPLE?"

Pay attention to your fellow students and current or potential colleagues. Do ask yourself if you feel like you're one of them, or if this feels right. This will help you decide which specialty of Medicine you want to go into. There is some truth to stereotypes, such as Family Medicine physicians being really patient, or Pediatricians being fun-loving. Make sure you feel at home with potential coworkers, since you will be spending the majority of your time with those kinds of people. Of course there are exceptions though, and you can be an exception, as well, and role model for others.

32. BE PREPARED TO WORK VERY LONG HOURS

You will be expected to study and work long hours during Medical School and Residency training, sometimes 80 hours per week or more. Consider that a full-time 9 to 5 job takes up only 40 hours per week. Normal labor law regulations do not apply in the field of Medicine, unfortunately. It was only recently that the 80 hour work-week restriction for Residency programs was created. Oftentimes, however, doctors take work home and just don't report it if they go past 80 hours out of fear of getting their Residency program into trouble, which could result in their program losing accreditation. Then they would have to scramble to find another one, which is a very difficult process (see #6).

The amount of information you need to learn is immense, and it is impossible to learn everything. This is why doctors specialize. Some Medical trainees have likened Medical learning to "trying to drink out of a fire hose." Information will be thrown at you at a rapid pace, and it becomes overwhelming if you expect to be able to absorb it all.

33. ASSESS YOUR TIME-MANAGEMENT SKILLS

Because of the long work hours, most doctors in training do not get enough nutrition, sleep, exercise, or ability to nurture or maintain their relationships with friends and family. Many struggle to keep up with household tasks, such as laundry and cleaning. It is even harder to be a parent during this brutal training path. Be honest about your time-management skills. If you struggle with efficiency, try to improve in that area, or ask for help.

Efficiency matters not only outside of the job, but also while you're on the job. Depending on your field, you will have to see a huge number of patients per day, on average in the 20s but some places can see up to 60. Oftentimes appointment slots are only 10-15 minutes long, which is not enough time to gather information, especially on complex patients, build a connection, or do a thorough exam. Part of the appointment also needs to be spent taking vitals, administering vaccines, or doing other tasks. Good communication and coordination among the medical assistants, nurse, and other members of the team are vital, and the best clinics run like well-oiled machines. Inpatient settings (hospitalized patients) allow a bit more flexibility, but you usually need to have seen and examined all your assigned patients and be prepared to present/talk about them to your team on "Morning Rounds" by 8-9 AM every day. Many doctors report feeling overwhelmed by this unrelenting pace and volume. They feel more like "assembly-line" factory workers than the compassionate healers they hope to be. Many become exhausted and start to see patients more as cases than humans. As the patient population grows (i.e. people are becoming sicker due to the obesity epidemic, and also living longer due to medical advances), and doctor shortages become greater, this pressure to see and do more will become even more relentless.

34. BE PREPARED TO WORK ODD, IRREGULAR HOURS

There's no getting around it; the Medical training path will affect your sleep. You will have to work night shifts, sometimes for a whole month or two in a row, 5 to 6 nights per week. Sometimes you will have to work 24-hour shifts (which can extend up to 28 hours). There are usually no scheduled breaks or chances to nap. Years ago, there were no hour restrictions at all, and doctors worked 72-hour shifts and over 100 hours per week.

35. CHECK HOW YOU HANDLE SLEEP DEPRIVATION

If you cannot function without good sleep or a regular sleep schedule, Medical training will be very difficult for you. Research has shown that driving sleep-deprived is the same as driving drunk. Many doctors have suffered mental breakdowns, seizures, hallucinations, or car accidents from sleep deprivation. This is extremely dangerous, but due to the huge demands of hospitals needing to care for patients 24/7, this work culture is unlikely to change anytime soon.

36. BE AWARE OF HIGH MALPRACTICE RATES

Unfortunately, the U.S. has high rates of malpractice lawsuits. In a capitalist society where "the customer is always right," many patients have unrealistic expectations of their doctors, who are only human and WILL make mistakes occasionally. As a result, doctors have had to learn defensive Medicine, documenting everything in detail, because their notes may get scrutinized and picked apart later by lawyers. This can happen many years after the incident as well, since each state and situation has different statutes of limitations. For Obstetricians for example, a child they deliver may be later found to have an issue related to the delivery. Even if this is found several years later, the parents can still file a lawsuit, up until age 18 of the child.

37. YOU WILL LIKELY SPEND MORE TIME WITH A COMPUTER, THAN WITH PATIENTS

Because of the need for thorough defensive documentation, doctors' notes have become increasingly longer. Technological advances have also moved notes to electronic form (Electronic Medical Records, or EMRs) instead of written notes, which have their own unique systems' issues. There are often boxes to click and nuances to fill out that force a doctor to either spend many extra hours of their free time on paperwork, or try to document while they're in the room with the patient. When they have to see so many patients each hour and only have 5-10 minutes with them, there simply isn't time to do work outside of the rooms, or the alternative is to stay very late or take work home, which many doctors do. Very few doctors are able to consistently stay on time.

Most doctors spend more time on documentation and other paperwork such as filling out forms, reviewing records, and coordinating care, than on actual patient contact. There are sadly more and more encounters where patients report doctors look more at their computer screens than at them, which interferes with the human connection, the very reason many people went into Medicine in the first place.

38. MEDICAL DOCUMENTATION IS UNNECESSARILY COMPLEX

There is an unnecessarily vast number of different EMRs, thus there is always a learning curve for each particular system. The original goal was to have records be more legible, accessible, and easily shared between doctors, such as when patients move to different locations and change doctors. Unfortunately, this was not accomplished, because the EMRs are so different and do not communicate well among each other. As a result, information can get lost if patients see different doctors with different systems. They usually have to fax paper records from one office to another since they cannot use the same EMR software. Because of competition between the different EMRs, there will not be a unifying EMR system anytime soon, though doctors are petitioning and speaking out about this flaw.

39. YOU WILL NOT HAVE AS MUCH AUTONOMY AS YOU'D LIKE

The other issue with the U.S. healthcare system is that it is intertwined with business. Pharmaceutical companies and insurance companies have sway over doctors' decisions, unfortunately. Some doctors feel pressured to order more tests in order to make more money for their clinics to stay running. Others have expressed frustration with the difficulties they encounter with ordering the tests they wanted for their patients because their patients' insurances did not cover them. Medical costs are insanely high without insurance in the United States. There are some exceptions, such as Medicare and the V.A. systems, but the majority of the population has to deal with this flawed general system.

This is something I feel we can learn from other countries' single-payer systems, such as Canada and Germany. Healthcare is a universal right, and should be affordable for everyone! An astounding 30% of people can't get the care they need due to insurance issues!!

Because of this, many people ignore their medical issues and delay seeking care or don't seek care at all. Their medical issues worsen and they then find themselves in an Emergency Room, whereas a simple office visit earlier could have prevented this. For example, Diabetes is a chronic disease of high blood sugar, but it has devastating effects on the eyes, kidneys, nerves, and skin's ability to heal from wounds. Diabetic medication is very expensive as well. If patients do not take care of their Diabetes, they can go blind, need toe amputations, kidney transplants or artificial kidneys, or even die.

40. YOU WILL HAVE MORE CONTROL OVER YOUR SCHEDULE ONCE YOU FULLY COMPLETE THE PATH

Once you have finally graduated Residency, you will have attained the status of a senior physician, called an "Attending" physician. You will have more control over your schedule and will not have to work 80 hours a week anymore, unless you choose to. You can start your own clinic or join a group. Some groups require you to be "on call" to cover patients during non-business hours. You can also take on part-time or temporary jobs such as Locum Tenens, and nowadays there are even location-independent opportunities in Telemedicine. You can also do the non-clinical jobs as well (see #16).

Practicing Medicine is extremely expensive. The Board certification exam is >$1000, and you need to retake them every 10 years. Each state's Medical licenses range from $150-1300 and last only 2 years, so they need constant renewal. You may also need a license to be able to prescribe controlled substances, such as strong opioid pain medications, known as a

DEA license, which is $731 for a 3-year period. You may also need other certifications depending on where you work, such as CPR for children (Pediatric Advanced Life Support).

41. YOU CAN WORK IN ACADEMIC OR PRIVATE PRACTICE

The two main types of Attending doctors are Academic and Private doctors. The Academic ones work with and teach Residents, Medical Students, and other trainees, and do research and other administrative tasks. The Private practice doctors focus solely on patient care. Some Residency programs set you up more for one route vs. the other, but you can switch between them as well. In general, Private practice doctors make more than Academic doctors, but it depends on the specific job.

Many people apply for Attending jobs during their last year of Residency, since the process can take a while. Applying for a Medical license can take up to 6 months to complete and may include fingerprinting, drug tests, and other tests to check if you've been adequately vaccinated against certain diseases.

Credentialing with a specific clinic or hospital can also take months and may require orientation events, etc. There is no Match system for Attending jobs; it is more like standard job applications. You may say no, and you may have many offers from several positions. You also do have the power to try to negotiate your salary.

42. YOU CAN ALSO DO A FELLOWSHIP FOR EVEN MORE TRAINING

After Residency, you can become even more specialized by doing a Fellowship, such as Gastroenterology (intestine doctor) or Oncology (cancer doctor) which takes 1-3 years, depending on the field. You get the same or slightly higher salary as a Resident's, and receive further training. The hours and workload can still be brutal, so the people who choose to do them are incredibly passionate about getting that further training. Internal Medicine (general care of adults) is the largest field for Residency and has the highest rates of Fellowships, in almost every organ system.

43. MENTAL HEALTH ISSUES AFFECT AT LEAST ONE-THIRD OF ALL DOCTORS

Perhaps Medicine's most well-kept secret is the effect it has on its workers. The training path is abusive because it deprives people of their basic human rights, such as enough hours to rest, sleep, eat, or take bathroom breaks. The high stress of seeing suffering and death so up close is also traumatic. We easily accept that war veterans return with Post-Traumatic Stress Disorder (PTSD), yet we don't recognize that doctors see the same horrors, sometimes worse. As a result, more than 33% of all doctors meet criteria for depression, even if they don't recognize or admit to it.

44. THE SYSTEM IS SLOW TO CHANGE

Unfortunately the current system does not admit to its flaws, and tries to push the blame and burden entirely onto its victims. Hospitals use terms such as "Burnout" and "Resiliency" to make doctors think that they themselves are at fault, that they are too weak to handle these pressures, when in reality anyone would suffer from these violations of basic human rights. They offer "Wellness" programs and lectures to teach doctors techniques to cope with stress, which can only help so much when doctors are not given adequate time or energy to implement them. A solution would be to hire more workers so that they can honor labor law restrictions, but many institutions do not have the funding or capacities to do so. Without recognition, these abusive systems are slow to change.

45. ANY WAVERING IS SEEN AS WEAKNESS

Medicine unfortunately has a toxic culture. There are extremely high expectations of doctors, since any mistake can result in harm to someone else, or even death. We forget sometimes that even doctors are only human too. Many doctors have perfectionistic, type A, hard-working personalities. They are hard on themselves and can carry the guilt and burdens of their mistakes for years. But they try to keep on a brave face, and don't want to be seen as weak, so they pretend everything is fine.

46. ASKING FOR HELP IS EXTREMELY DIFFICULT DUE TO STIGMA

Because of the stigma attached to mental health issues, it is extremely difficult and risky for doctors to reach out for help. Many licensing boards will refuse or revoke a doctor's right to practice Medicine if the doctor admits to even a long-ago history of depression or anxiety, even if they have been working for decades without any issues. Some are also forced to undergo random drug testing since mental health disorders increase someone's risk of abusing alcohol or drugs. Many doctors report that they don't feel like they can be completely honest, out of fear of these harsh consequences. As a result, this terrible culture of secrecy, stigma, and shame continues.

47. GOING TO ONE'S OWN APPOINTMENTS IS DIFFICULT

A doctor's schedule makes it extremely hard to take time for self-care. Many doctors report feeling like burdens to their colleagues if they ask someone to cover for them while they go to an appointment, so they just don't go and keep putting off their own health. Even though they are supposed to be models of health for their patients, very few doctors are actually taking good care of themselves. Mental health appointments have the added stress of being a black mark on a doctor's record, since licensing boards can demand to see all medical records of any doctor in question. This is why some doctors travel long distances, use fake names, and pay therapists or psychiatrists in cash for their services.

48. MEDICINE IS AN OCCUPATIONAL RISK FACTOR FOR SUICIDE

Worst of all, the mental health problem in Medicine is so severe that being a doctor statistically doubles your chances of committing suicide, compared to the average population or other jobs. This happens in all stages of the path, even those who have completed it but who still battle with the ongoing difficulties of Medicine, some systemic and some cultural. Dr. Pamela Wible (see Resources section below) has counted over 1,300 physician suicides since 1858, some completely unexpected from the most seemingly happy, successful, and well-adjusted of people. Doctors have suffered immensely and as a result have become very good at hiding their pain and focusing entirely on others (their patients). They become good at putting on masks. They often do not take the time or effort to think of themselves, and as a result, their health issues worsen, until one day they reach a breaking point.

49. YOU DON'T HAVE TO SUFFER SILENTLY

Times are changing for the better, but mental health is still not talked about enough. Even in the cases when someone committed suicide, their colleagues are expected to carry on working, without being able to take adequate time to grieve or process. Patients need to be seen, and work needs to be done.

This applies to any healthcare job, and there is a shortage of workers of all kinds including doctors, nurses, and health aides.

So many healthcare workers suffer silently, but you don't have to be one of them. If you need help, don't hesitate to reach out to someone. Don't wait until things get so bad for you that you can't do day-to-day tasks, or you start having thoughts of harming yourself or wanting it all to end.

50. CHECK IN WITH YOURSELF OFTEN

Many doctors, including myself, realized that Medicine is different from what we thought it was, and are trying to change it or at least bring awareness to the problems in this field. No matter what anyone tells you, it is completely okay to change your mind at any point if you feel that something feels off or isn't right for you; it is never too late. You have every right to explore and form your own opinions from your experiences, and make your own decisions. Don't be afraid to make a change for the sake of your health or happiness!

MY STORY:

I have experienced firsthand much of what I have written above. I went into Medicine without an adequate enough understanding of the field and all of its flaws and secrets.

My parents were both doctors, and I had grown up with this expectation that I would follow in their footsteps. I loved to draw and had always dreamt of becoming an artist/cartoonist as a child, but I had always felt obligated to consider Medicine as well. I applied to a combined College and Medical School program (Brown University/The Warren Alpert Medical School of Brown University) and was very torn when I received the acceptance letter. Aside from the expectations and pride from my family, I personally felt pressured to not waste this incredible opportunity that so many others would have died for. I reassured myself that I could opt out or leave at any time, so I thought I would try to make it fit.

Because I was already accepted into Medical School, I didn't allow myself to truly explore and figure out who I was in college, though I had inklings of my passions for writing, drawing cartoon/Japanese anime/manga-style, teaching, languages, psychology, sociology, and travel. I fortunately did not have to take the MCAT standardized test, but I still had to do all the Pre-Requisite "Pre-Med" classes. My greatest mistake was not taking time off to further explore myself, think, and try to decide if Medicine was right for me; I bowed my head down and walked onwards straight into Medical School, though Brown allowed up to a 2-year gap before Medical School while still saving my spot. I think I was afraid that if I took time off, I'd never return.

Medical School was okay for me. I was a decent test-taker, so I did not struggle with passing exams. I enjoyed talking to patients and hearing their stories, but did not care much for figuring out the mystery behind their symptoms and problems, which is the heart of being a doctor. I found it tolerable, but it did not pump passion through my veins, which I felt a true career calling should do. My astute advisor even asked me if I truly wanted to be a doctor, in my heart of hearts, because after every clinical rotation, I breathed a sigh of relief knowing that I could choose to never do that again by not picking that field. It became a problem when I reached the end of all my rotations and did not really want to pick a single one to train in for Residency.

Because of my passion for women's equality and reproductive rights, I decided I could do the most good as an Obstetrician/Gynecologist, a doctor who focused solely on caring for women through a wide range of their life experiences, from giving birth to going through menopause. I entered Residency and Match Day with trepidation, some part of me wishing I had not "Matched" so I could escape from this path.

I did Match, however, and I walked into Residency with excitement and cautious optimism since many people had told me that Residency is "better" than Medical School because you will actually be a true doctor caring for patients, rather than an extra member of the team. (Medical Students were primarily there to learn, and while could be incredibly helpful, were never essential to a team's functioning).

However, I found that this heightened level of responsibility terrified me. I had always been a perfectionistic overachiever, someone who was hard on myself for mistakes, and I had naively thought I could over-prepare for each patient (like I had for tests) and never make mistakes. When I found out that this is simply not possible, I began to realize the true weight of a doctor's responsibility. I thankfully never made a mistake causing grave harm or death to a patient, but I knew it was inevitable if I continued on this path.

One particular event is burned into my memory. I was observing a vaginal birth of a baby who was feet-first. Normally babies are delivered head-first because the head is the largest part of the body and once it is delivered past the cervix (opening of the womb), the rest of the body usually smoothly follows. However, sometimes the baby is not facing head-down, and in these cases, doctors usually decide on delivering via Cesarean Section (C-Section, a surgery to cut open the womb through the abdomen). This was an emergency situation in which the baby's lower body was already partially out, so the delivery had to be continued vaginally. However, the head became stuck for several agonizing minutes, and the baby suffocated to death. The mother also suffered immensely since she did not have enough pain-numbing medications, and I will never forget her blood-curdling cries of pain and suffering.

It was then that I realized that I would not be able to live with myself if I were the doctor in that situation. Why did I have to stay in a field where people could, and likely would, die by my hand? That doctor did nothing wrong; sometimes bad events just happen. As powerful as humans are, we cannot prevent all tragedies. I spoke with others to grieve and process this traumatic event, but did not allow myself to admit that I would have benefited from seeking more professional help. I did not want to bother my overworked colleagues, and tried to push on.

The realization of a doctor's role stayed with me, however. And as I saw and did more deliveries of babies, I started to realize I was in a very high-risk field. I knew this going in, but I don't think I truly understood it until after that event. It took me some time to decide since I had become good at compartmentalizing and ignoring my feelings this entire time, but I ultimately decided to leave for a lower risk field (Family Medicine). I also sought more work-life balance since Obstetricians continued to deliver babies at irregular times of day and night and were frequently on long calls.

Family Medicine was definitely a better fit for me. I enjoyed talking to patients and forming relationships, so as their primary physician, I was the one out of all their doctors who knew them best. Still, I found that my creativity was stifled and I wasn't experiencing enough gratification in my day-to-day life due to the documentation, insurance, and malpractice issues, which all took away from the experience of connecting with patients. These issues permeate all stages of Medicine, even as an Attending doctor. There are some revolutionary doctors who have started their own clinics and unique systems of patient care (see Dr. Pamela Wible and Dr. ZDoggMD in the Resources section below), but the vast majority of doctor jobs are confined to 15-minute appointments, limitations imposed by insurance companies, and all the other issues above (#36-39).

I heard life would get "better" as an Attending physician compared to a Resident's, but I had also heard the same about Residency vs. Medical School, and that was definitely not true for me. Limiting the amount of time spent in toxicity is better than nothing, but that does not solve the underlying problems.

I also took matters into my own hands for the first time and spoke with many Attending doctors about their experiences, feelings, and regrets, something I wish I had done in high school or even earlier. I spoke with people who pursued non-clinical fields and those who kept up their Medical backgrounds part-time. I found out about Dr. Pamela Wible and learned even more about how flawed and abusive the Medical system is, and how widespread mental health suffering and suicides are among doctors.

After gaining a better understanding through my own firsthand experiences and investigations, I was able to make a fully informed decision. I decided to listen to my heart, which had been protesting for a long time, though I had become too disconnected with myself to hear it. I had tried so hard to make a Medical career fit. I asked myself why was I not satisfied with such a noble career? I was already here and had finally jumped through all the hoops! Why couldn't I just be happy carrying on this path, as I had for my past 30 years of existence?

I want to help change the system by bringing awareness to it and de-stigmatizing mental health issues. Medicine treats its trainees horribly, and part of me left because I refuse to be a part of its system of abuse. The other part of me wanted to nurture the other, buried parts of myself, nearly lost in the all-consuming fire of Medical training.

I am now doing part-time Telemedicine to help people access affordable and confidential mental healthcare, one of my missions, and I aim to join another Telemedicine movement to prescribe birth control remotely to help women all over the world take control of their lives and careers. Occasionally I take on part-time Locum Tenens assignments to fill in for other doctors who are on leave or in need of a break themselves. I also blog about my experiences, coach others on how to break free from suboptimal paths and mindsets, and create educational cartoon drawings teaching about women's health and other issues such as boundaries, consent, and self-esteem, all while traveling the world learning from other cultures. My life's mission is to bring us all closer together in mutual understanding, respect, and acceptance of one another, and to help each and every person live out their best lives—healthy, balanced, and true to their hearts. I'm a huge believer in holistic health and addressing the mental, emotional, and spiritual aspects, not just physical health.

Though I probably would not do it again if I could turn back time, I am immensely grateful for all my experiences. My Medical background has challenged me and taught me the true meanings of empathy, perseverance, self-awareness, and strength. Though I am starting on different paths now much later than most, those years were not wasted. If I can help even one person avoid the same mistakes I made, I would be overjoyed. I was afraid to listen to my heart until many years later, out of fear and ignorance, and I would be so humbled if I can help others learn or find inspiration from my story.

Thank you so much for reading my book! I'm happy to chat with you anytime. Please reach out to me via my blog or at LTnomad@outlook.com.

OTHER HELPFUL RESOURCES

"What I've Learned From 1300 Doctor Suicides." Pamela Wible MD.

https://www.idealMedicalcare.org/ive-learned-547-doctor-suicides/

"Medical Satire with a Health 3.0 Mission." Dr. Zubin Damania aka ZDoggMD

https://zdoggmd.com/

For Applying to Medical Schools:

https://students-Residents.aamc.org/advisors/help-your-advisees-apply-Medical-school/

https://students-Residents.aamc.org/choosing-Medical-career/article/free-resources-every-aspiring-physician-should-rea/

http://med.stanford.edu/md/student-affairs/student-wellness/_jcr_content/main/panel_builder_2/panel_1/download_1095234323/file.res/Roadmap%20to%20Choosing%20a%20Medical%20Specialty%20.pdf

For Applying to Residencies:

https://students-Residents.aamc.org/applying-Residency/applying-Residencies-eras/tools-Residency-applicants/

https://www.ecfmg.org/echo/us-Residency-application-process.html

https://freida.ama-assn.org/Freida/#/

For Changing Residencies:

https://students-Residents.aamc.org/applying-Residency/findaResident/

http://www.Residentswap.org/how_it_works.php

READ OTHER 50 THINGS TO KNOW BOOKS

50 Things to Know to Get Things Done Fast: Easy Tips for Success

50 Things to Know About Going Green: Simple Changes to Start Today

50 Things to Know to Live a Happy Life Series

50 Things to Know to Organize Your Life: A Quick Start Guide to Declutter, Organize, and Live Simply

50 Things to Know About Being a Minimalist: Downsize, Organize, and Live Your Life

50 Things to Know About Speed Cleaning: How to Tidy Your Home in Minutes

50 Things to Know About Choosing the Right Path in Life

50 Things to Know to Get Rid of Clutter in Your Life: Evaluate, Purge, and Enjoy Living

50 Things to Know About Journal Writing: Exploring Your Innermost Thoughts & Feelings

50 Things to Know

Stay up to date with new releases on Amazon:
https://amzn.to/2VPNGr7

Mailing List: Join the 50 Things to Know Mailing List to Learn About New Releases

50 Things to Know

Please leave your honest review of this book on Amazon and Goodreads. We appreciate your positive and constructive feedback. Thank you.

Made in the USA
Middletown, DE
11 May 2020